How to Grow Your Medical Practice by Certifying Patients on the Georgia Low THC Oil Registry

BRIAN L. PONDER, ESQ.

Copyright © 2019 Brian L. Ponder, Esq.

All rights reserved.

ISBN: 9781692144135

DEDICATION

This book is dedicated to my late grandmother, Rubye Blanche Bess Hollis.

TABLE OF CONTENTS

	Acknowledgments	i
1	Introduction	Pg 3
2	Definitions	Pg 5
3	Georgia's Hope Act	Pg 19
4	Qualifying Medical Conditions	Pg 25
5	How to Certify Patients	Pg 31
6	Legal Do's and Don'ts	Pg 49
7	Who will produce low THC oil	Pg 57
8	Who will sell low THC oil	Pg 65
9	Branding & Marketing	Pg 71
10	Marketing Company v. Employees	Pg 83
	Appendix	Pg 85

ACKNOWLEDGMENTS

Thanks "Q" (Creative eGenius) for your hard work!

1 INTRODUCTION

This book is for physicians and healthcare systems that want to grow their medical practices by certifying qualified patients on the Georgia Low THC Oil Registry. On April 17, 2019, Governor Brian Kemp (R) signed HB324, Georgia's Hope Act, into law. The law took effect on July 1, 2019.

Georgia's Hope Act allows qualified patients in Georgia to access medical cannabis oil with no more than 5% THC by weight, known as "low THC oil." Also, six (6) private growers to produce low THC oil, along with two (2) designated universities: University of Georgia and Fort Valley State University.

HOW TO GROW YOUR MEDICAL PRACTICE BY CERTIFYING PATIENTS ON THE GEORGIA LOW THC OIL REGISTRY

The Georgia State Board of Pharmacy will develop rules and regulations for dispensing low THC oil and issue dispensing licenses to specialty pharmacies and retail outlets that will be located throughout Georgia.

There were approximately 9,500 low THC oil cardholders when the law was signed in April 2019. The population of Georgia is now over 10.5 million. With the addition of "intractable pain" as a qualifying condition for a low THC oil registration card and the increase in patients seeking alternative, non-opioid pain relief, it is estimated that the number of patients seeking low THC oil will grow exponentially fast. There are thirteen (13) qualifying medical conditions. This presents a huge opportunity for physicians and healthcare systems to meet the demand by treating patients with the qualifying conditions and certifying patients who seek access to low THC oil on the Georgia Low THC Oil Registry. As a result, you can grow your medical practice in this new industry.

2 DEFINITIONS

The terms below are unique to Georgia's Hope Act. Familiarize yourself with these terms and definitions.

- **"Applicant"** means a corporate entity applying for a license.
- **"Available capital"** means corporate assets that are available to fund business operations.
- **"Board"** means the Georgia Composite Medical Board.
- **"Cardholder"** means the person identified on a "Low THC Oil Permit" as being authorized to possess low THC oil. A cardholder may be an eligible patient or a caregiver.
- **"Caregiver"** means the parent, guardian, or

legal custodian of an individual who is less than 18 years of age or the legal guardian of an adult.

- **"CBD"** means cannabidiol.
- **"Class 1 production license"** mean a license to produce and manufacture low THC oil, limited to growing only in an indoor facility up to 100,000 square feet of cultivation space.
- **"Class 2 production license"** means a license to produce and manufacture low THC oil, limited to growing only in an indoor facility up to 50,000 square feet of cultivation space.
- **"Commission"** means the Georgia Access to Medical Cannabis Commission.
- **"Condition"** means:
  - (A) **Cancer**, when such disease is diagnosed as end stage or the treatment produces related wasting illness or recalcitrant nausea and vomiting;

- (B) **Amyotrophic lateral sclerosis (ALS** or **Lou Gehrig's disease)**, when such disease is diagnosed as severe or end stage;
- (C) **Seizure disorders** related to a diagnosis of epilepsy or trauma related head injuries;
- (D) **Multiple sclerosis (MS)**, when such disease is diagnosed as severe or end stage;
- (E) **Chrohn's disease**;
- (F) **Mitochondrial disease**;
- (G) **Parkinson's disease**, when such disease is diagnosed as severe or end stage;
- (H) **Sickle cell disease**, when such disease is diagnosed as severe or end stage;
- (I) **Tourette's syndrome**, when such

syndrome is diagnosed as severe;
- (J) **Autism spectrum disorder**, when such disorder is diagnosed for a patient who is at least 18 years of age, or severe autism, when diagnosed for patient who is less than 18 years of age;
- (K) **Epidermolysis bullosa**;
- (L) **Alzheimer's disease**, when such disease is diagnosed as severe or end stage;
- (M) **Acquired immune deficiency syndrome** (**AIDS**), when such syndrome is diagnosed as severe or end stage;
- (N) **Peripheral neuropathy**, when such symptoms are diagnosed as severe or end stage;
- (O) **Post-traumatic stress disorder** (**PTSD**) resulting from direct exposure

to or the witnessing of a trauma for a patient who is at least 18 years of age; or
- o (P) **Intractable pain**.
- **"Department"** means the Georgia Department of Public health.
- **"Designated universities"** means the University of Georgia and Fort Valley State University.
- **"Designated university license"** means a license issued by the commission to a designated university to produce, manufacture, and purchase low THC oil.
- **"Dispense"** means to sale or provision of low THC oil to registered patients by a dispensing licensee.
- **"Dispensing license"** means a specialty license issued by the State Board of Pharmacy or commission to dispense low THC oil to registered patients.

HOW TO GROW YOUR MEDICAL PRACTICE BY CERTIFYING PATIENTS ON THE GEORGIA LOW THC OIL REGISTRY

- **"DPH"** means department of public health.
- **"Eligible patient"** means a resident of Georgia who has been certified by a physician licensed by and in good standing with the Georgia Composite Medical Board as having on a qualifying Condition.
- **"Intractable pain"** means pain that has a cause that cannot be removed and for which, according to accepted medical practice, the full range of pain management modalities appropriate for the patient has been used for a period of time of at least six months without adequate results or with intolerable side effects.
- **"Grow"** means cultivating and harvesting cannabis for use in producing low THC oil.
- **"Licensee"** means any business, or owner of such business, with a valid production license.
- **"Low THC oil"** means an oil that contains CBD and not more than 5% THC by weight.

- **"Low THC Oil Patient Registry"** means the database maintained by the Department of all eligible patients and their caregivers on whose behalf applications for a Low THC Oil Permit have been submitted and approved by the Department.
- **"Manufacture"** means to process cannabis to produce low THC oil.
- **"Minority"** means an individual who is a member of a race which comprises less than 50 percent of the total population of the state.
- **"Minority business enterprise"** means a small business concern which is owned and controlled by one or more minorities and is authorized to do and is doing business under the laws of Georgia, paying all taxes duly assessed, and domiciled within Georgia.
- **"Owned and controlled"** means a business:
    - (A) Which is at least 51 percent owned by

one or more minorities or, in the case of a publicly owned business, at least 51 percent of all classes or types of the stock is owned by one or more minorities; and
    - (B) Whose management and daily business operations are controlled by one or more minorities.
- **"Owner"** means any person who directly or indirectly owns, actually or beneficially, or controls 5 percent or greater of interests of the applicant or any licensee. In the event that one person owns a beneficial right to interests and another person holds the voting rights with respect to such interests, then both shall be considered an owner of such interests.
- **"Physician"** means an individual licensed to practice medicine in the State of Georgia.
- **"Product"** means low THC oil delivered through an oil, tincture, transdermal patch,

lotion or capsule, but not including any food products infused with low THC oil, including, but not limited to, cookies, candies, or edibles.

- **"Registered patient"** means an individual who is legally authorized to possess and use low THC oil pursuant to Code Section 31-2A-18.

- **"Registry"** means the Low THC Oil Patient Registry.

- **"Tracking system"** means a seed-to-sale tracking system to track marijuana that is grown, processed, manufactured, transferred, stored, or disposed of and low THC oil that is transferred, stored, sold, dispensed, or disposed of.

HOW TO GROW YOUR MEDICAL PRACTICE BY CERTIFYING PATIENTS ON THE GEORGIA LOW THC OIL REGISTRY

HOW TO GROW YOUR MEDICAL PRACTICE BY CERTIFYING PATIENTS ON THE GEORGIA LOW THC OIL REGISTRY

NOTES

HOW TO GROW YOUR MEDICAL PRACTICE BY CERTIFYING PATIENTS ON THE GEORGIA LOW THC OIL REGISTRY

NOTES

HOW TO GROW YOUR MEDICAL PRACTICE BY CERTIFYING PATIENTS ON THE GEORGIA LOW THC OIL REGISTRY

NOTES

HOW TO GROW YOUR MEDICAL PRACTICE BY CERTIFYING PATIENTS ON THE GEORGIA LOW THC OIL REGISTRY

NOTES

3 GEORGIA'S HOPE ACT

On April 17, 2019, Governor Brian Kemp (R) signed Georgia's Hope Act (HB 324) into law, which took effect on July 1, 2019. Georgia's Hope Act allows patients to legally access medical cannabis oil in Georgia with no more than 5% THC level by weight. The law allows up to six (6) private growers to cultivate medical cannabis oil preparations, along with two (2) designated universities: University of Georgia and Fort Valley State University. Qualified patients will be allowed to obtain low THC oil from licensed specialty pharmacies and retail dispensaries.

The Georgia Access to Medical Cannabis Commission is duly created under Georgia's Hope Act to license and regulate medical cannabis growers.

HOW TO GROW YOUR MEDICAL PRACTICE BY CERTIFYING PATIENTS ON THE GEORGIA LOW THC OIL REGISTRY

Per the law, the Commission shall consist of seven (7) members who shall be appointed as follows:

- Three (3) member appointed by the Governor;
- Two (2) members appointed by the Lieutenant Governor;
- Two (2) members appointed by the Speaker of the House of Representatives.

Commission members shall serve four-year terms. The Governor shall designate one of his or her appointees as the chairperson. The Commission shall meet upon the call of the chairperson or upon the request of three (3) members. Any vacancy on the Commission shall be filled for the unexpired term by appointment by the original appoint authority. Members of the Commission shall serve without compensation, but shall receive the same expense allowance per day as that received by a member of the General Assembly for each day in a meeting.

NOTES

HOW TO GROW YOUR MEDICAL PRACTICE BY CERTIFYING PATIENTS ON THE GEORGIA LOW THC OIL REGISTRY

NOTES

HOW TO GROW YOUR MEDICAL PRACTICE BY CERTIFYING PATIENTS ON THE GEORGIA LOW THC OIL REGISTRY

NOTES

HOW TO GROW YOUR MEDICAL PRACTICE BY CERTIFYING PATIENTS ON THE GEORGIA LOW THC OIL REGISTRY

NOTES

4 QUALIFYING MEDICAL CONDITIONS

Georgia's Hope Act lists the following sixteen (16) medical conditions and diseases for patients to qualify for the Georgia Low THC Oil Registry card:

1. **Cancer**, when such disease is diagnosed as end stage or the treatment produces related wasting illness or recalcitrant nausea and vomiting;
2. **Amyotrophic lateral sclerosis (ALS or Lou Gehrig's disease)**, when such disease is diagnosed as severe or end stage;
3. **Seizure disorders** related to a diagnosis of epilepsy or trauma related head injuries;
4. **Multiple sclerosis (MS)**, when such disease is diagnosed as severe or end stage;
5. **Chrohn's disease**;

6. **Mitochondrial disease**;

7. **Parkinson's disease**, when such disease is diagnosed as severe or end stage;

8. **Sickle cell disease**, when such disease is diagnosed as severe or end stage;

9. **Tourette's syndrome**, when such syndrome is diagnosed as severe;

10. **Autism spectrum disorder**, when such disorder is diagnosed for a patient who is at least 18 years of age, or severe autism, when diagnosed for patient who is less than 18 years of age;

11. **Epidermolysis bullosa**;

12. **Alzheimer's disease**, when such disease is diagnosed as severe or end stage;

13. **Acquired immune deficiency syndrome (AIDS)**, when such syndrome is diagnosed as severe or end stage;

14. **Peripheral neuropathy**, when such

symptoms are diagnosed as severe or end stage;

15. **Post-traumatic stress disorder (PTSD)** resulting from direct exposure to or the witnessing of a trauma for a patient who is at least 18 years of age; or

16. **Intractable pain.**

HOW TO GROW YOUR MEDICAL PRACTICE BY CERTIFYING
PATIENTS ON THE GEORGIA LOW THC OIL REGISTRY

NOTES

HOW TO GROW YOUR MEDICAL PRACTICE BY CERTIFYING PATIENTS ON THE GEORGIA LOW THC OIL REGISTRY

NOTES

HOW TO GROW YOUR MEDICAL PRACTICE BY CERTIFYING PATIENTS ON THE GEORGIA LOW THC OIL REGISTRY

NOTES

5 HOW TO CERTIFY PATIENTS

Physicians licensed in Georgia may certify patients for Georgia Low THC Oil registration cards, after first registering themselves on the Georgia Low THC Oil Registry. The Georgia Low THC Oil Registry is established and maintained by the Georgia Department of Public Health. Registration is free.

Physician registration onto the Georgia Low THC Oil Registry is done online. The physician would create a username, which will be an email address, and a password, and provide the following information: license number and expiration date, DEA number, first, middle initial, and last name, date of birth, last 4 digits of physician's social security number, mailing address, telephone, and fax number.

HOW TO GROW YOUR MEDICAL PRACTICE BY CERTIFYING PATIENTS ON THE GEORGIA LOW THC OIL REGISTRY

Physicians may submit registration applications on behalf of their patient and their caregivers. Specific information will be required for input, including:

a. Name, address, and date of birth of the patient;

b. Name, address, and Georgia license number of the physician providing the certification;

c. The medical condition or conditions that make the patient eligible for the Low THC Oil Registry;

d. How long the patient has been a resident of Georgia;

e. Whether the certifying physician has a doctor-patient relationship with the patient; and

f. Whether the certifying physician is treating the patient for the medical condition or conditions that make the patient eligible for the Low THC Oil Registry.

HOW TO GROW YOUR MEDICAL PRACTICE BY CERTIFYING PATIENTS ON THE GEORGIA LOW THC OIL REGISTRY

The Georgia Department of Public Health has developed two (2) requires forms to certify patients: (1) a "Low THC Oil Waiver" form that must be completed and signed in the presence of a notary; and (2) a "Physician Certification Form" must be completed and signed by the certifying physician. Also, the Georgia Department of Health has a physician user guide on using the registration portal. Download free copies of these forms here:

www.ga-hope.com/forms

Georgia law completely protects health care institutions and providers from registering patients. Section 51-1-29.6 of the Official Code of Georgia provides, "A health care institution shall not be subject to any civil liability, penalty, licensing sanction, or other detrimental action and a health care provider shall not be subject to any civil liability, penalty, denial of a right or privilege, disciplinary action by a professional licensing board, or other detrimental action for allowing an individual or caregiver to possess, administer, or use low THC oil on the premises of a health care institution or offices of a health care provider, provided that the possession of such substance is in accordance with the laws of this state." Further, Section 16-12-231 of the Official Code of Georgia exempts physicians from arrest, prosecution, or penalty, namely stating, "The following persons and entities, when acting in accordance with the provisions of this article, shall not be subject to arrest, prosecution, or any civil or administrative penalty, including a civil penalty or disciplinary action by a professional licensing board, or be denied any right or privilege, for the medical use, prescription, administration, manufacture, or distribution of low THC oil:

(1) A registered patient who is in possession of

an amount of low THC oil authorized under Code Section 16-12-191 or such patient's caregiver, parent, or guardian;

(2) A physician who certifies a patient to the Department of Public Health as being diagnosed with a condition or in a hospice program and authorized to use low THC oil for treatment pursuant to Code Section 31-2A-18;

(3) A pharmacist or pharmacy that dispenses or provides low THC oil to a registered patient;

(4) The commission or its employees or contractors associated with the production of low THC oil in accordance with this article; and

(5) A designated university, an employee of a designated university, or any other person associated with the production of low THC oil in accordance with this article."

HOW TO GROW YOUR MEDICAL PRACTICE BY CERTIFYING PATIENTS ON THE GEORGIA LOW THC OIL REGISTRY

Physicians should feel secure in certifying qualified patients to legally access low THC oil in Georgia.

Physicians may register on the Georgia Low THC Oil Registry on the Georgia Department of Public Health's Georgia Low THC Oil Registry portal. Physician's may use the following link to access it:

www.ga-hope.com/register

Registered physicians may access the portal here:

www.ga-hope.com/portal

Once a patient is approved by the physician, the waiver and certifications forms are completed, and the patient is entered into the Low THC Oil Registry, a "Low THC Oil Registry" card will be issued. Patients are notified when their card is ready for pickup within about fifteen (15) business days.

Patients will have the option to pick up their card at any one (1) of the twenty (20) public health offices throughout Georgia, and must present valid ID and pay a $25 for the card at the time of pick up. The registration card is valid for two (2) years from issuance or until death, whichever happens first.

A map of card pickup locations can be found here:

www.ga-hope.com/cards

Below is a list of the twenty (20) public health offices throughout Georgia where patients may pick up their low THC oil registration cards once available:

1. **State Office of Vital Records**,
    1680 Phoenix Blvd., #100
    Atlanta, GA 30349
    (404) 679-4702

HOW TO GROW YOUR MEDICAL PRACTICE BY CERTIFYING PATIENTS ON THE GEORGIA LOW THC OIL REGISTRY

2. **Bibb County Health Department**
   171 Emery Hwy.
   Macon, GA 31217
   (478) 745-0411

3. **Carrol County Health Department**
   1004 Newnan Rd.
   Carrollton, GA 30116
   (770) 836-6667

4. **Chatham County Health Department**
   1395 Eisenhower Dr.
   Savannah, GA 31406
   (912) 356-2441
   or
   1602 Drayton St.
   Savannah, GA 31401
   (912) 651-3378

5. **Cherokee County Health Department**

   1219 Univeter Rd.

   Canton, GA 30115

   (770) 345-7371

   or

   7545 Main St., #100

   Woodstock, GA 30188

   (770) 928-0133

6. **Clarke County Health Department**

   345 N. Harris St.

   Athens, GA 30601

   (706) 389-6921

   or

   410 McKinley Drive

   Athens, GA 30601

   (706) 369-5816

7. **Cobb County Health Department**

   1650 County Services Pkwy.

   Marietta, GA 30008

   (770) 514-2300

8. **Colquitt County Health Department**

   214 W. Central Ave.

   Moultrie, GA 31768

   (229) 589-8464

9. **Decatur County Health Department**

   928 S. West St.

   Bainbridge, GA 39819

   (229) 248-3055

10. **DeKalb County Health Department**

    445 Winn Way

    Decatur, GA 30030

    (404) 294-3700

11. **Fulton County Health Department**
10 Park Place South, SE
Atlanta, GA 30303
(404) 613-1205

12. **Hall County Health Department**
1290 Athens St.
Gainesville, GA 30507
(770) 531-5600

13. **Laurens County Health Department,**
654 County Farm Rd., Dublin, Ga 31021,
(478) 272-2051

14. **Lowdnes County Health Department**
206 S. Patterson St.
Valdosta, GA 31601
(229) 333-5257

15. **Muscogee County Health Department**

    2100 Comer Ave.

    Columbus, GA 31904

    (706) 321-6300

16. **Richmond County Health Department**

    950 Laney-Walker Blvd.

    Augusta, GA 30901

    (706) 721-5900

17. **Sumter County Health Department**

    1601 N. Martin Luther King Blvd.

    Americus, GA 31719

    (229) 924-3637

18. **Troup County Health Department**
900 Dallis St.
LaGrange, GA 30240
(706) 845-4085

19. **Ware County Health Department**
604 Riverside Ave.
Waycross, GA 31501
(855) 473-4374

20. **Whitfield County Health Department**
800 Professional Blvd.
Dalton, GA 30720
(706) 279-9600

Replacements for an unexpired Low THC Oil cards that have been lost or damaged may be ordered by the certifying physician. The fee replacement cards is $25.

NOTES

HOW TO GROW YOUR MEDICAL PRACTICE BY CERTIFYING PATIENTS ON THE GEORGIA LOW THC OIL REGISTRY

NOTES

NOTES

NOTES

HOW TO GROW YOUR MEDICAL PRACTICE BY CERTIFYING PATIENTS ON THE GEORGIA LOW THC OIL REGISTRY

6 LEGAL DO'S AND DON'TS

There are some legal do's and don'ts that should be considered in dealing with low THC oil in Georgia. Several laws apply specifically to Georgia physicians.

DO register on the Georgia Low THC Oil Registry in order to submit applications for patients.

DON'T submit applications for patients that you do not have a doctor-patient relationship with and are treating for a qualifying condition under the law.

DO stay up to date with the rules and regulations related to Georgia's Hope Act. At the publishing of this book, the members of the Georgia Access to Medical Cannabis Commission has not been appointed yet, and the Georgia Board of Pharmacy has not released dispensing rules and regulations.

HOW TO GROW YOUR MEDICAL PRACTICE BY CERTIFYING PATIENTS ON THE GEORGIA LOW THC OIL REGISTRY

Subscribe to the GHC blog for updates:

www.ga-hope.com/blog

DON'T be surprised at the number of patients that will inquire about the benefits of low THC oil and how they may qualify to obtain a registration card. As news develop about the possible benefits of low THC oil, patients will begin inquire about it.

DO provide registered patients with information of licensed low THC oil dispensaries, upon request.

DON'T allow low THC oil licensees to directly advertise or market to your patients as it is unlawful. Section 16-12-215(b) of the Official Code of Georgia provides, "No licensee shall advertise or market low THC oil to registered patients or the public; provided, however, that a licensee shall be authorized to provide information regarding its low THC oil directly to physicians."

HOW TO GROW YOUR MEDICAL PRACTICE BY CERTIFYING PATIENTS ON THE GEORGIA LOW THC OIL REGISTRY

DO study medical literature regarding the use, benefits, and efficacy of low THC oil use by patients.

DON'T have a financial interest in a Georgia low THC oil licensee, if you are a certifying physician. Section 16-22-224(b) of the Official Code of Georgia provides, "No physician who certifies individuals to the commission pursuant to Code Section 31-2A-18 for use of low THC oil to treat certain conditions shall own, operate, have a financial interest in, or be employed by a low THC oil manufacturer or distributor, including any licensee under this part. This subsection shall not prohibit a physician from furnishing a registered patient or his or her caregiver, upon request, with the names of low THC oil manufactures or distributors. Any physician violating this Code section shall be guilty of a misdemeanor."

DO submit reports to the Georgia Medical Board. Section 31-2A-18(e) of the Official Code of Georgia provides, "The board shall require physicians to issue semiannual reports to the board. Such reports shall require physicians to provide information, including, but not limited to, dosages recommended for a particular condition, patient clinical responses, levels of tetrahydrocannabinol or tetrahydrocannabinolic acid present in test results, compliance, responses to treatment, side effects, and drug interactions. Such reports shall be used for research purposes to determine the efficacy of the use of low THC oil as a treatment of conditions."

DON'T produce, grow, manufacture, or dispense low THC oil or products. Section 16-12-201 of the Official Code of Georgia provides, "Except as otherwise provided in this article, it shall be unlawful for any person in this state to produce, grow, manufacture, or dispense low THC oil or any products related to its production in this state."

HOW TO GROW YOUR MEDICAL PRACTICE BY CERTIFYING PATIENTS ON THE GEORGIA LOW THC OIL REGISTRY

NOTES

HOW TO GROW YOUR MEDICAL PRACTICE BY CERTIFYING
PATIENTS ON THE GEORGIA LOW THC OIL REGISTRY

NOTES

HOW TO GROW YOUR MEDICAL PRACTICE BY CERTIFYING PATIENTS ON THE GEORGIA LOW THC OIL REGISTRY

NOTES

HOW TO GROW YOUR MEDICAL PRACTICE BY CERTIFYING PATIENTS ON THE GEORGIA LOW THC OIL REGISTRY

NOTES

7 WHO WILL PRODUCE LOW THC OIL

The Commission may issue two (2) classes of low THC oil production licenses:

(i) two (2) Class 1 production licenses and

(ii) four (4) Class 2 production licenses.

A Class 1 production licensee shall be authorized to:

(1) grow cannabis only in indoor facilities for use in producing low THC oil, limited to 100,000 square feet of cultivation space and

(2) manufacture low THC oil. Class 1 production license applicants must be a Georgia entity with a bank account in Georgia.

Class 1 license applicants must submit proof that it has at least $2 million in cash reserves and their plans. The nonrefundable application fee is $25,000; if approved, the initial license fee is $200,000, and upon annual renewal, the license renewal fee is $100,000.

A Class 2 production licensee shall be authorized to:

(1) grow cannabis only in indoor facilities for use in producing low THC oil, limited to 50,000 square feet of cultivation space and

(2) manufacture low THC oil.

Class 2 production license applicants must be a Georgia entity with a bank account in Georgia. Class 2 production license applicants must submit proof that it has at least $1.25 million in cash reserves and their plans. The nonrefundable application fee is $5,000; if approved, the initial license fee is $100,000, and upon annual renewal, the license renewal fee is $50,000.

Class 1 and Class 2 production licensees must be

HOW TO GROW YOUR MEDICAL PRACTICE BY CERTIFYING PATIENTS ON THE GEORGIA LOW THC OIL REGISTRY

operation within 12 months of their respective award dates or their license will be revoked. Also, no person or entity can hold an interest in more than one license at any one time. Ownership interests in more than one license at any one time shall be cause for revocation of all licenses. The Commission will select licensees via a competitive application process.

HOW TO GROW YOUR MEDICAL PRACTICE BY CERTIFYING PATIENTS ON THE GEORGIA LOW THC OIL REGISTRY

NOTES

NOTES

NOTES

NOTES

HOW TO GROW YOUR MEDICAL PRACTICE BY CERTIFYING PATIENTS ON THE GEORGIA LOW THC OIL REGISTRY

8 WHO WILL SELL LOW THC OIL

Pharmacies and retail outlets will sell low THC oil. The Georgia State Board of Pharmacy is charged with developing an annual, nontransferable specialty dispensing license for pharmacies and retail outlets to dispense low THC oil to registered patients. Further, the Georgia State Board of Pharmacy will develop rules and regulations regarding dispensing pharmacies and retail outlets in the state of Georgia. At the time of the publishing of this book, no dispensary licenses have been issued, nor have any rules or regulations been promulgated by the Georgia State Board of Pharmacy. The GHC blog will post updates.

HOW TO GROW YOUR MEDICAL PRACTICE BY CERTIFYING
PATIENTS ON THE GEORGIA LOW THC OIL REGISTRY

When available, you may find dispensary locations at:

www.ga-hope.com/oil

NOTES

HOW TO GROW YOUR MEDICAL PRACTICE BY CERTIFYING PATIENTS ON THE GEORGIA LOW THC OIL REGISTRY

NOTES

HOW TO GROW YOUR MEDICAL PRACTICE BY CERTIFYING PATIENTS ON THE GEORGIA LOW THC OIL REGISTRY

NOTES

NOTES

9 BRANDING & MARKETING

Physicians can expand their patient base by branding their practice as one specializing in the treatment of the various qualifying conditions for low THC oil and marketing to that patient population in Georgia.

Physicians with their own practices face challenges that include not only quality patient care, but growing the practice, paying the rent, utilities and insurance. The costs to run a medical practice can be very high. Maintaining a steady flow of patients is very important in order to have a thriving practice. However, to do this takes specialized work and effort. Namely, getting your name out there to prospective patients is a common challenge. However, it does not have to be an impossible feat.

HOW TO GROW YOUR MEDICAL PRACTICE BY CERTIFYING PATIENTS ON THE GEORGIA LOW THC OIL REGISTRY

Grow your practice via branding and marketing. Branding identifies your specific practice area. Marketing gets your brand to your patient base. Combine branding and marketing to grow a practice. Also, the type of brand you create and the type of marketing that you do will determine your results. With proper branding and marketing, your practice can be distinguished from others and be in the front of prospective patients for them to contact you.

There are several considerations that should go into your branding and marketing campaign. This book will discuss the various mediums and resources.

Podcast Development. The public wants information on-demand. Mainstream radio is almost completed replaced by online podcast broadcasts. Almost half of the homes in the U.S. listen to podcasts. Podcasts are a tool giving physicians an opportunity to give potential patients information about themselves and their respective practice areas.

A great app to produce a podcast is Anchor (**anchor.fm**). Download Anchor in your app store. Anchor allows you to publish your podcast across all major podcasting sites with one click of a button. The app can record a podcast with numerous people as easily as making a phone call. This app is FREE.

Website Development. It is critical to develop your medical practice's online identity via a website. You want to capture your target patient base visually. You want to do this by creating a memorable impression for prospective patients on your website. It is essential to have a website that is operable on any device, that is, a computer or a mobile phone. Your medical practice needs to develop a responsive website that looks great on any browser, device, or screen size. A good custom website could easily cost $2,000 (on the low end), not including changes.

A custom website is the most professional option. It is highly advised not to cut costs here. However, if resources cannot support a web developer, then online website builders can be a good viable option. Using an online website builder is one of the fastest ways to set up a website. Many available platforms provide simple, drag and drop tools that make creating a website simple and very straightforward. Not all website builder platforms are created equal. Some are more reliable and flexible than others.

<u>10 popular website builders are:</u>

(1) wix.com,

(2) constantcontact.com,

(3) site123.com,

(4) jimbo.com,

(5) squarespace.com,

(6) godaddy.com,

(7) wordpress.com,

(8) weebly.com,

(9) webs.com,

(10) web.com.

HOW TO GROW YOUR MEDICAL PRACTICE BY CERTIFYING PATIENTS ON THE GEORGIA LOW THC OIL REGISTRY

Local Search. People no longer need to look at a phone directory or phone book to find a doctor. Most of the time, people search for doctors online. People will typically resort to a quick Google search. Developing a robust online presence is essential for being visible and outranking colleagues online. Develop a digital footprint by building consistent and quality listings for your practice, so your practice can be found anywhere by patients who are looking for you.

Below are six (6) popular local search sites:
1. Yelp 9yelp.com)
2. Google+ Local (google.com/business/)
3. Bing Local (bingplaces.com)
4. Yahoo! Local (smallbusiniess.yahoo.com/local)
5. Foursquare (foursquare.com)
6. Facebook (facebook.com)

HOW TO GROW YOUR MEDICAL PRACTICE BY CERTIFYING PATIENTS ON THE GEORGIA LOW THC OIL REGISTRY

In your local search listings, be sure to include your (i) full business name and logo, (ii) physical address, (iii) hours of operation, and (iv) parking availability.

SEO. SEO stands for search engine optimization. Search engines are used to post ads online. Therefore, SEO is critical to gain visibility online. Customized search engine optimization campaigns can position your practice brand to appear directly in from of prospective patients that are looking for treatment providers online. SEO experts can inspect your website to ensure it is set up properly to rank high organically. A competitive analysis can be done in order to recommend a tailored marketing strategy for your medical practice.

Reputation Management. Prospective patients do no trust what a practice says about itself online, thanks to the rise and popularity of online reviews. With this in mind, it is important to create a customized review management campaign to bolster your practice's reputation online. This will make a good digital first impression to potential patients.

Eight (8) of the best online reputation tools are:
1. Awario (awario.com)
2. Reputology (reputology.com)
3. GoFish Digital Complaint Search (gofishdigitial.com/complaint-search/)
4. SEO SpyGlass (link-assistant.com/seo-spyglass/)
5. Grade.us (grade.us)
6. Brandwatch (brandwatch.com)
7. ReviewTrackers (reviewtrackers.com)
8. IFTTT (ifttt.com)

Photography/Videography. Creating a photoshoot, or video or your practice and staff can positively impact your practice's image. Showcase the values and culture of your brand, so that your practice does not get lost in the sea of practices. Use professional photography and videography.

HOW TO GROW YOUR MEDICAL PRACTICE BY CERTIFYING PATIENTS ON THE GEORGIA LOW THC OIL REGISTRY

Social Media. Social media is in everyone's hand. Therefore, a robust social media campaign is more important now than ever before for your practice. Your practices services need to be posted daily! However, most practices do not have the time or knowledge of how to effectively do so. Frequently post quality content on your social media account daily and optimize customer searches with hasghtags.

The top three (3) social media sites that you definitely want to have a presence online with your practice are:

1. Facebook (Facebook.com)
2. Instagram (Instagram.com)
3. Twitter (Twitter.com)

Post helpful and informative content and run ads.

Graphic Design. Most practices do not think about the importance of graphic design in their practice. However, you want to use the best illustrative tools in maintain freshness of your brand.

Accordingly, you want to develop persuasive images using graphic design on your website and brochures. You can hire good graphic designers on sites such as Fiverr (**fiverr.com**) and Upwork (**upwork.com**).

SEM/PPC. SEM means search engine marketing and PPC stands for pay-per-click. SEM is a form of internet marketing that involves the promotion of websites by increasing their visibility in search engine results pages (SERPSs) primarily through paid advertising. Basically, SEM is the process of gaining website traffic by purchasing ads on search engines. PPC is a model of internet marketing in which advertisers pay a fee each time one of their ads is clicked. Essentially it is a way of buying visits to your website, rather than trying to get visits organically.

Marketing Automation. Marketing is one of the major elements of running a business, including a medical practice. However, handling all the tasks that come with your business while keeping up with the demands of modern marketing can be complicated and exhausting. This is why marketers and businesses opt to implement marketing automation software. Email marketing is great, but marketing automation takes email marketing to the next level. Technology allows you to track your web traffic, how visitors navigate through your website, time spent on webpages, and even how your prospective patients found you online. Marketing automation literally will do the work for you by interacting with your leads.

According to online reports, below are the reported top twenty (20) marketing automation software companies of 2019:

1. HubSpot Marketing (hubspot.com)
2. Pardot (pardot.com)
3. SendinBlue Email (sendinblue.com)
4. SharpSpring (sharpspring.com)
5. EngageBay (enginebay.com)
6. GrowSurf (growsurf.com)

7. bpm'online marketing (bpmonline.com)
8. Marketo (marketo.com)
9. Active Campaign (activecampaign.com)
10. LeadSquared Marketing Automation (leadsquared.com)
11. iContact Pro (icontact.com)
12. Wishpond (wishpond.com)
13. Infusionsoft (keap.com)
14. Boomtrain (zetaglobal.com)
15. Optimizely (Optimizely.com)
16. NAVIK MarketingAl (absolutdata.com/analytics-products/navik-converter-marketing/)
17. Percolate (percolate.com)
18. IBM Marketing Cloud (ibm.com/case-studies/ibm-marketing-cloud)
19. AdRoll (adroll.com)
20. ContactPigeon (contactpigeon.com)

Targeted Social Media Ads. You can target any demographic that correlates with the profile of your prospective patients. You can create targeted ads appear the same as natural posts from trusted family members and friends, strategically placed in prospective patients' social media feed.

App Development. Popular brands have an app. Develop an app that can showcase your practice area. Your app needs to work on both Android and iOS. Utilize app technology to scale your medical practice. You can hire good app developers on websites such as Fiverr (fiverr.com) and Upwork (upwork.com).

Print Media. Your medical practice only has one chance to make a first impression to future patients. Your practice's business card and brochures need to be like a firm handshake. Leave your prospective patient impressed with unforgettable graphics. Use physical media like brochures to leave a stunning imprint of your brand on your prospects' mind.

10 MARKETING COMPANY & EMPLOYEES

You must decide whether to use a marketing company or hire employees, or both, to do your medical practice's branding and marketing work. Each have their own unique benefits, pros, and cons.

First, hiring an employee has some benefits. Namely, you have control over the employee's time. However, you are responsible for wages, insurance, taxes, etc., which are the basic liabilities of an employer. An experienced marketing manager with 10-19 years of experience earns an average total compensation of $75,574 per year in Georgia. In their late career (20 years and higher), employees earn an average total compensation of $90,985. This does not include any applicable taxes and insurance, etc.

Second, hiring a marketing company has great benefits without employee-related liabilities and costs. First, you have control of costs with a marketing company as you can set a budget and pick and choose the level of services that you want to have. Second, you get to shop around for the most quality company and get the most competitive pricing. Third, considering the costs, taxes, insurance, and other liabilities associated with employing persons, outsourcing your branding and marketing can be more cost-effective in the long run. Most practices do not employ marketing staff, as that is just not an arena that a practice can commit to focus on. Therefore, small or large, most medical practices engage the use of marketing companies to maximize the return on their marketing dollars, so they can focus on what they do best: medicine.

For information about branding & marketing your practice, go to **www.ga-hope.com/marketing**.

APPENDIX

(Contacts and Resources)

GEORGIA HOPE CONSULTANTS, INC.

2221 Peachtree Road NE, Suite X10

Atlanta, Georgia 30309

Telephone: (404) 969-3055

Facsimile: (404) 420-2856

Website: www.ga-hope.com

Service: Complete solutions for Georgia's low THC oil industry, serving licensees, vendors, and physicians.

GEORGIA DEPARTMENT OF PUBLIC HEALTH

2 Peachtree Street, NW

15th Floor

Atlanta, Georgia 30303-3186

Telephone: (404) 657-2700

Website: www.dph.georgia.gov/low-thc-oil-registry

HOW TO GROW YOUR MEDICAL PRACTICE BY CERTIFYING PATIENTS ON THE GEORGIA LOW THC OIL REGISTRY

GEORGIA COMPOSITE MEDICAL BOARD

2 Peachtree Street, NW

6th Floor

Atlanta, Georgia 30303-3465

Telephone: (404) 656-3913

Facsimile: (404) 656-9723

Email: medbd@dch.ga.gov

Website: medicalboard.georgia.gov

GEORGIA STATE BOARD OF PHARMACY

2 Peachtree Street, NW

6th Floor

Atlanta, Georgia 30303

Telephone: (404) 651-8000

Facsimile: (470) 386-6137

Website: gbp.georgia.gov

NOTES

NOTES

NOTES

NOTES

HOW TO GROW YOUR MEDICAL PRACTICE BY CERTIFYING
PATIENTS ON THE GEORGIA LOW THC OIL REGISTRY

NOTES

HOW TO GROW YOUR MEDICAL PRACTICE BY CERTIFYING PATIENTS ON THE GEORGIA LOW THC OIL REGISTRY

NOTES

HOW TO GROW YOUR MEDICAL PRACTICE BY CERTIFYING PATIENTS ON THE GEORGIA LOW THC OIL REGISTRY

NOTES

NOTES

HOW TO GROW YOUR MEDICAL PRACTICE BY CERTIFYING
PATIENTS ON THE GEORGIA LOW THC OIL REGISTRY

NOTES

HOW TO GROW YOUR MEDICAL PRACTICE BY CERTIFYING PATIENTS ON THE GEORGIA LOW THC OIL REGISTRY

NOTES

ABOUT THE AUTHOR

Brian L. Ponder, Esq. is a graduate of Northwestern University (B.A.) and Southern University Law Center (J.D.). Ponder is a civil trial attorney, entrepreneur, and founder, president, and CEO of Georgia's Hope Consultants, Inc. ("GHC"). GHC is headquartered in Atlanta, Georgia, and provides complete solutions for the Georgia Low THC Oil industry. GHC serves the needs of Class 1 and Class 2 production license applicants and licensees, pharmacy and retail outlet dispensary license applicants and licensees, vendors to production and dispensary licensees, and helps certifying physicians and healthcare systems with medical practice branding and marketing. Find GHC online at **www.ga-hope.com**.

www.ingramcontent.com/pod-product-compliance
Lightning Source LLC
Chambersburg PA
CBHW070425220526
45466CB00004B/1540